THE TREE OF LIFE

PHYSICAL REGENESIS

First Edition 1917
George Washington Carey

New Edition 2018
Edited by Tarl Warwick

COPYRIGHT AND DISCLAIMER

FOREWORD

This present text is one of the stranger works (of a corpus of quite strange works!) written in its era. The result of George Washington Carey's spiritual efforts, it expounds the theory (then in some degree of vogue) that the organ systems, cells, and chemistry of the human body overlaps with the Christian religion. In that era, a common claim was made that the human body seemingly correlating with biblical symbolism could not be coincidental and that it should be categorized and used to govern the human condition- usually individually, unfortunately sometimes as a collective.

Shunning sexual intercourse, alcohol consumption, excessive eating, and war, Carey likens the pores and sweat to a steam powered system venting its gas, and ruminates on the brain in general and especially the pineal gland, even categorizing twelve inorganic chemical materials to the twelve signs of the zodiac according to their closeness to traditional astrology's explanation of the character of the signs. These chemical materials, themselves inorganic, found in the human cell, fascinated the burgeoning late pre-modern occult, along with its less demon-friendly but equally superstitious christian counterparts searching to perfect mankind, cure disease, and bring forth the post-revelational utopia of New Jerusalem.

This edition of "The Tree of Life" has been edited to modernize some language and improve format. Care has been taken to retain all original intent and meaning.

THE TREE OF LIFE

INTRODUCTION

What Jehovah, Eve, David, and John Say

"And Jehovah God commanded the man saying: Of every tree in the garden thou mayest freely eat: but of the tree of the knowledge of good and evil, thou shalt not eat of it, for the day that thou eatest thereof, thou shalt surely die. And the woman said unto the serpent, 'Of the fruit of the trees of the garden we may eat: but of the fruit of the tree which is in the midst of the garden, God hath said, Ye shall not eat of it, neither shall ye touch it, lest ye die.' "Gen. 1:16.

"And he shall be like a tree planted by the streams of water, that bringeth forth its fruit in its Season, whose leaf also does not wither, and whatsoever he doeth shall prosper." David in Psalm I.

"And on this side of the river and on that was the tree of life bearing twelve manner of fruits, yielding its fruit every month: And the leaves of the tree were for the healing of the Nations." John the Revelator, Chapt. 22.

PART ONE

Wonders and Possibilities of the Human Body

The human race has been asleep, and has dreamed that property and money are the true wealth of a nation, sacrificing men, women and children to the chimerical idea that danced in visionary splendor through their brains. The result of this is to be seen in the uneasiness that prevails everywhere. But humanity is

4

waking up, slowly but surely and beginning to realize that it, itself, is the most precious thing on earth.

The old-established statement that the individuals that make up the race are imperfect is no more true than that a pile of lumber is imperfect, that is to be afterward reformed or built into a house. As it is the carpenter's business to take the lumber, which is perfect as material, and build the house, so it is the legitimate work of spiritual man to take the perfect material everywhere present and build, by the perfect law of chemistry and mathematics, the perfected, harmonious human being, and with this material, employ the same law to build up society collectively. It is a well-known physiological fact that the blood is the basic material of which the human body is continually built. As is the blood, so is the body; as is the body, so is the brain; as is the brain, so is the quality of thought. As a man is built, so thinks he.

According to the views of students of modern alchemy, the Bible both the Old and New Testaments are symbolical writings, based primarily upon this very process of body building. The word Alchemy really means Fleshology. It is derived from Chem, an ancient Egyptian word, meaning flesh. The word Egypt also means flesh, or anatomy. Alchemy, however, in its broader scope, means the science of solar rays. Gold may be traced to the Sun's rays. The word gold means solar essence. The transmutation of gold does not mean the process of making gold, but does mean the process of changing gold, solar rays, into all manner of materialized forms, vegetable, mineral, etc. The ancient alchemist studied the process of Nature in her operations from the volatile to the fixed, the fluid to the solid, the essence to the substance, or the abstract to the concrete, all of which may be summed up in the changing of spirit into matter. In reality, the alchemist did not try to do anything. He simply tried to search out nature's processes in order that he might

5

comprehend her marvelous operations.

To be sure, language was used that to us seems symbolical and often contradictory, but it was not so intended, nor so at all in reality. We speak in symbols. If a man is in delirium, caused by alcohol in his brain-cells, we say he has "snakes in his boots." Of course, no one supposes that the words are to be taken literally. Yet if our civilization should be wiped out, and our literature translated after four or five thousand years, those who read our history might be puzzled to know what was meant by "snakes in his boots."

Again, it has been believed by most people that the words, "transmutation of base metals into gold," used by alchemists, referred to making gold. But a careful study of the Hebrew Cosmogony, and the Kabala, will reveal the fact that the alchemist always referred to solar rays when he used the word gold. "Base metals," simply means matter, or basic. The dissolving, or disintegration of matter, the combustion of wood or coal, seemed as wonderful to these philosophers as the growth of wood or the formation of coal or stone. So, the transmutation of base metals into gold simply meant the process of changing the fixed into the volatile, or the dematerialization of matter, either by heat or chemical process.

It is believed by modern students of alchemy that the books of the Old and New Testaments are a collection of alchemical and astrological writings, dealing entirely with the wonderful operation of aerial elements (Spirit) in the human body, so fearfully and wonderfully made. The same authority is given for the statements, "Know ye not that your bodies are the temple of the living God" and "Come unto me all ye that labor and are heavy laden and I will give ye rest." According to the method of reading the numerical value of letters by the Kabala, M and E figure B, when united. Our B is from the Hebrew Beth, meaning a house or temple the temple of the soul the body. Thus by coming into the realization that the body is really the Father's House, temple of God, the soul secures peace and contentment or rest.

The human body is composed of perfect principles, gases, minerals, molecules, or atoms; but these builders of flesh and bone are not always properly adjusted.

The planks or bricks used in building houses may be endlessly diversified in arrangement, and yet be perfect material.

Solomon's temple is an allegory of man's temple the human organism. This house is built (always being built) "without sound of saw or hammer." The real Ego manifests in a house, beth, church, or temple i. e., Soul-of-Man's Temple. The solar (soular) plexus is the great central Sun or dynamo on which the Subconscious Mind (another name for God) operates and causes the concept of individual consciousness. The brain of man is the Son of God, the mediator (medium) between the central dynamo and the Cosmic Ocean of Space.

Thus digestion or combustion of food, circulation of blood, inbreathing the breath of life (aerial elements), is carried on by the co-operation of the Holy Trinity; God, the solar plexus; the Son, the brain; and the Holy (whole) Spirit, or air. No wonder that the seers and alchemists of old declared that "Your bodies are the temple of the living God" and "The kingdom of Heaven is within you." But man, blinded by selfishness, searches here and there, scours the heavens with his telescope, digs deep into earth, and dives into ocean's depths, in a vain search for the Elixir of Life that may be found between the soles of his feet and the crown of his head. Really our human body is a miracle of mechanism. No work of man can compare with it in accuracy of its process and the simplicity of its laws. At maturity, the human skeleton contains about 165 bones, so delicately and perfectly adjusted that science has despaired of ever imitating it. The muscles are about 500 in number; length of alimentary canal, 32 feet; amount of blood in average adult, 30 pounds, or one-fifth the weight of the body; the heart is six inches in length and four inches in diameter, and beats seventy times per minute, 4200 times per hour, 100,800 per day, 36,720,000 per year. At each beat, two and one-half ounces of blood are thrown out of it, 175 ounces per minute, 656 pounds per hour, or about eight tons per day.

All the blood in the body passes through the heart every three minutes; and during seventy years it lifts 270,000,000 tons of blood.

The lungs contain about one gallon of air at their usual degree of inflation. We breathe, on an average, 1200 breaths per hour; inhale 600 gallons of air, or 24,000 gallons daily. The aggregate surface of air-cells of the lungs exceed 20,000 square inches, an area nearly equal to that of a room twelve feet square. The average weight of the brain of an adult is three pounds, eight ounces; the average female brain, two pounds, four ounces. The convolutions of a woman's brain cells and tissues are finer and more delicate in fiber and mechanism, which evidently accounts for the intuition of women. It would appear that the difference in the convolutions and fineness of tissue in brain matter is responsible for the degrees of consciousness called reason and intuition. The nerves are all connected with the brain directly, or by the spinal marrow, but nerves receive their sustenance from the blood, and their motive power from the solar plexus dynamo. The nerves, together with the branches and minute ramifications, probably exceed ten millions in numbers.

The skin is composed of three layers, and varies from one-eighth to one-quarter of an inch in thickness. The average area of skin is estimated to be about 2000 square inches. The atmospheric pressure, being fourteen pounds to the square inch, a person of medium size is subject to a pressure of 40,000 pounds. Each square inch of skin contains 3500 sweat tubes, or perspiratory pores (each of which may be likened to a little drain tile) one-fourth of an inch in length, making an aggregate length of the entire surface of the body 201,166 feet, or a tube for draining the body nearly forty miles in length.

Our body takes in an average of five and a half pounds of food and drink each day, which amounts to one ton of solid and liquid nourishment annually, so that in seventy years a man eats and drinks 1000 times his own weight.

There is not known in all the realms of architecture or mechanics one little device which is not found in the human organism. The pulley, the lever, the inclined plane, the hinge, the "universal joint," tubes and trap-doors; the scissors, grind-stone, whip, arch, girders, filters, valves, bellows, pump, camera, and Aeolian harp; and irrigation plant, telegraph and telephone systems all these and a hundred other devices which man thinks he has invented, but which have only been telegraphed to the brain from the Solar Plexus (cosmic center) and crudely copied or manifested on the objective canvas.

No arch ever made by man is as perfect as the arch formed by the upper ends of the two legs and the pelvis to support the weight of the trunk. No palace or cathedral ever built has been provided with such a perfect system of arches and girders. No waterway on earth is so complete, so commodious, or so populous as that wonderful river of life, the "Stream of Blood." The violin, the trumpet, the harp, the grand organ, and all the other musical instruments, are mere counterfeits of the human voice. Man has tried in vain to duplicate the hinges of knee, elbow, fingers and toes, although they are a part of his own body.

Another marvel of the human body is the self-regulation process by which nature keeps the temperature in health at 98 degrees. Whether in India, with the temperature at 130 degrees, or in the arctic regions, where the records show 120 degrees below the freezing point, the temperature of the body remains the same, practically steady at 98 degrees, despite the extreme to which it is subjected.

It was said that "all roads lead to Rome." Modern science has discovered that all roads of real knowledge lead to the human body. The human body is an epitome of the universe; and when man turns the mighty searchings of reason and investigation within that he has so long used without the New Heaven and Earth will appear. While it is true that flesh is made by a precipitation of blood, it is not true that blood is made from food. The inorganic or cell-salts contained in food are set free by the process of combustion or digestion, and carried into the circulation through the delicate absorbent tubes of the mucous membranes of stomach and intestines. Air, or Spirit, breathed into the lungs, enters the arteries (air carriers) and chemically unites with the mineral base, and by a wonderful transformation creates flesh, bone, hair, nails, and all the fluids of the body. On the rock (Peter or Petra, meaning stone) of the mineral salts is the human structure built, and the grave, stomach, or hell shall not prevail against it.

The minerals in the body do not disintegrate or rot in the grave. The fats, albumen, fibrine, etc., that compose the organic part of food, are burned up in the process of digestion and transposed into energy or force to run the human battery. Blood is made from air; thus all nations that dwell on earth are of one blood, for all breathe one air. The best food is the food that burns up quickest and easiest; that is, with the least friction in the human furnace. The sexual functions of man and woman; the holy operation of creative energy manifested in male and female; the formation of life germs in ovum and sex fluids; the Divine Procedure of the "word made flesh" and the mysteries of conception and birth are the despair of science.

"Know ye not that your bodies are the temple of the living God?" for "God breathed into man the breath of life."

In the words of Epictitus, "Unhappy man, thou bearest a god about with thee, and knowest it not."

Walt Whitman sings:

"I loaf and invite my soul; I lean and loaf at my ease, observing a spear of summer grass. Clear and sweet is my soul, and clear and sweet is all that is not my soul."

"Welcome every organ and attribute of me, and of any man hearty and clean, not an inch, not a particle of an inch, is vile, and none shall be less familiar than the rest."

"Divine am I, inside and out, and I make holy whatever I touch or am touched from."

"I say no man has ever yet been half devout enough; none has ever yet adored or worshiped half enough; none has begun to think how divine he himself is, and how certain the future is."

The vagus nerve, so named because of its wandering (vagrant) branches, is the greatest marvel of the human organism. Grief depresses the circulation, through the vagus, a condition of malnutrition follows, and tuberculosis, often of the hasty type, follows. The roots of the vagus nerve are in the medulla oblongata, at the base of the small brain or cerebellum, and explains why death follows the severing of the medulla. It controls the heart action, and if a drug such as aconite be administered, even in small doses, its effect upon this nerve is shown in slowing the action of the heart and decreasing the blood pressure. In larger doses it paralyzes the ends of the vagus in the heart, so that the pulse becomes suddenly very rapid and at the same time irregular. Branches of the vagus nerve reach the heart, lungs, stomach, liver and kidneys.

Worry brings on kidney disease, but it is the vagus nerve, and especially that branch running to the kidneys which under undue excitement or worry, or strain, brings about the paralysis of the kidneys in the performance of their functions. When we say that a man's heart sinks within him for fear or apprehension, it is shown by the effect of this nerve upon the heart action. If his heart beats high with hopes, or he sighs for relief, it is the vagus nerve that has conducted the mental state to the heart and accelerated its action or caused that spasmodic action of the lungs which we call a sigh.

The nerves of the human body constitute the "Tree of Life," with its leaves of healing. The flowing waters of the Rivers of Life are the veins and arteries through which sweep the red, magnetic currents of Love of Spirit made visible.

> Acids and alkalis acting,
> Proceeding and acting again,
> Operating, transmuting, fomenting,
> In throes and spasms of pain
> Uniting, reacting, atoning,
> Like souls passing under the rod
> Some people call it Chemistry,
> Others call it GOD.

THE TREE OF LIFE

Behold the divine telegraph system, the million nerve wires running throughout the wondrous temple, the temple not made with hands, the temple "made without sound of saw or hammer." View the Central Sun of the human system the Solar Plexus vibrating life abundantly.

Around this dynamo of God, you may see the Beasts that worship before the Throne day and night saying, "Holy, holy, art Thou, Lord God Almighty." The Beasts are the twelve plexuses of nerve centers, telegraph stations, like unto the twelve zodiacal signs that join hands in a fraternal circle across the gulf of space. Aviation, liquefied air, deep breathing for physical development and the healing of divers diseases rule the day. In every brain there are dormant cells, waiting for the "coming" of the bridegroom, the vibration of the air age (the Christ) that will resurrect them. Everywhere we have evidence of the awakening of dormant brain cells. Much, if not all, of spiritual phenomena, multiple personality, mental telepathy, and kindred manifestations, are explainable upon the hypothesis of the possibility of awakening and bringing into use of dormant brain cells.

The eye is hardly less wonderful, being a perfect photographer's camera. The retina is the dry plate on which are focused all objects by means of the crystalline lens. The cavity behind this lens is the shutter. The eyelid is the drop shutter. The draping of the optical dark room is the only black membrane in the entire body. This miniature camera is self-focusing, self-loading and self-developing, and takes millions of pictures every day in colors and enlarged to life size.

Charts have been prepared; marvelous charts which go to show that the eye has 729 distinct expressions conveying us many distinct shades of meaning. The power of color perception is overwhelming. To perceive red the retina of the eye must receive 395,000 vibrations in a second; for violet it must respond to 790,000,000. In our waking moments our eyes are bombarded every minute by at least 600,000,000 vibrations. The ear is a colossal mystery, and the phenomenon of sound is a secret only recorded in the Holy of Holies of the Infinite Mind. And what is mind?

We know absolutely nothing about it. Some believe that mind is the product of the chemical operation of matter, namely; the atoms or materials that compose the human body. These persons contend that all electrons are particles of pure Intelligence and know what to do. Others hold to the theory that universal Mind (whatever it may be) forms a body from some material, they know not what, and then plays upon it or operates through it.

> Visions of beauty and splendor,
> Forms of a long-lost race,
> Sounds and faces and voices
> From the fourth dimension of space ;
> And on through the universe boundless,
> Our thoughts go, lightning-shod ;
> Some call it Imagination,
> And others call it GOD!

We wonder and adore in the presence of that pulsing orb, the heart. Tons of the water of life made red by the Chemistry of Love sweep through this central throne every day, and flow on to enrich the Edenic Garden until its waste places shall bloom and blossom as the rose. Take my hand and go with me to the home of the Soul that wonderful brain. Can you count the whirling, electric, vibrating cells? No, not until you can count the sand grain on the ocean's shore. These rainbow-hued cells are the keys that the fingers of the soul strike to play its part in the Symphony of the Spheres.

THE TREE OF LIFE

At last we have seen the "Travail of the Soul and are satisfied." No more temples of the Magi now, but instead the Temple of the Ego, the glorious human Beth. At least we have found the true church of God, the human body. In this body, or church, spirit operates like some wizard chemist or electrician. No more searching through India's jungles or scaling the Himalayan heights in search for a master a mahatma or ancient priest dwelling in some mysterious cave where occult rites and ceremonies are supposed to reveal the wisdom of the past. But instead, you have found the Kingdom of the Real within the Temple that needs no outer Sun by day nor Moon nor Stars by night to lighten it. And then the enraptured Soul becomes conscious that the stone has been rolled away from the door of material concept where it has slept, and it now hears the voice of the Father within saying, "Let there be light!" and feels the freedom that comes with knowing that Being is one.

And now, man, the Ego, also realizes the meaning of the "Day of Judgment." It realizes that Judgment means understanding, hence the ability to judge. Man then judges correctly, for he sees the Wisdom of Infinite Life in all men, in all things, all events, and all environments. Thus does the new birth take place, and the Kingdom of Harmony reigns now. Man must realize, however, that he is the creator or builder of his own body, and that he is responsible for every moment of its building, and every hour of its care. He alone can select and put together the materials provided by the universe for its construction.

Man has been able to scale the heavens, to measure the distances between the stars and planetary bodies, and to analyze the component parts of suns and worlds, yet he cannot eat without making himself ill; he can foretell eclipses and tides for years in advance, but cannot look far enough ahead in his own affairs to say when he may be brought down with la grippe, or to calculate accurately the end of any bodily ill that may afflict him.

THE TREE OF LIFE

When he finds out what he really is, and how much he has always had to do in the making of himself what he is, he will be ready to grasp some idea of the wonderful possibilities of every human soul and body, and will know how completely and entirely is every man his own savior. Just so long as he denies his own powers, and looks outside of himself for salvation from present or future ills, he is indeed a lost creature. If the race is to be redeemed, it must come as the result of thought followed by action. If the race is to think differently than at present, it must have new bodies with new brains. Man must be born again.

Modern physiologists know that our bodies are completely made over every year, by the throwing off of worn-out cells and the formation of new ones, that is going on every minute. Nature will take care of the making-over process, but we are responsible for the plan of reconstruction. Man must learn to run the machinery of his body with the same mathematical accuracy as he now displays in control of an engine or automobile, before he can lay claim to his divine heritage and proclaim himself master of his own.

The law of life is not a separate agent working independently of mankind and separate from individual life. Man himself is a phase of the great law in operation. When he once fully awakens to the universal cooperation of the attributes and thoughts through which the great dynamic operates or proceeds, he the Ego one of the expressions of infinity, will be enabled to free himself from the seeming environments of matter, and thus realizing his power, will assert his dominion over all he has been an agent in creating. And he has indeed assisted in creating manifesting all that is. Being a thought, an exhalation of universal spirit, he is co-eternal with it. In material concept, we do not begin to realize the extent of our wisdom. When we awaken to spirit, consciousness knowledge that we are egos that have bodies or temples, and not bodies that have souls, or spirits, we see the object or reason of all symbols or manifestation, and begin to realize our own power over all created things.

And in this Aquarian age, great changes in nature's laws will be speedily brought to pass, and great changes in the affairs of humanity will result. The laws of vibration will be mastered, and through their operation material manifestations will be shaped and molded to man's will. It is only a matter of time when all the necessities of life will be produced directly from the elements of the air. It is well known by chemists that all manner of fruits, grains and vegetables are produced directly from the elements in air, and not from soil. The earth, of course, serves as a negative pole and furnishes the mineral salts of lime, magnesium, iron, potassium, sodium and silica, which act as carriers of water, oil, fibrin, sugar,etc., and thus build up the plant; but oil, sugar, albumin, etc., are formed by a precipitation or condensation of principles in air, and not from soil. This is a fact abundantly proved.

Mr. Berthelot, a scientist of France, Tesla, the Austrian wizard, and our own Edison have long held that food can be produced by a synthetic process from its elements artificially.

Some six or seven extracts, as well as coloring material, are now being manufactured in this manner. Madder is made almost exclusively by this process now. Sugar has recently been made in the laboratory from glycerin, which Professor Berthelot first made direct from synthetic alcohol. Commerce has now taken up the question; and an invention has been patented by which sugar is to be made upon a commercial scale, from two gases, at something like one cent per pound. M. Berthelot declares he has not the slightest doubt that sugar will eventually be manufactured on a large scale synthetically, and that the culture of sugar cane and beet root will be abandoned, because they have ceased to pay.

17

THE TREE OF LIFE

The chemical advantages promised by M. Berthelot to future generations are marvelous. He cites the case of alzarin, a compound whose synthetic manufacture by chemists has destroyed a great agricultural industry. It is the essential commercial principle of the madder root, which was once used in dyeing. The chemists have now succeeded in making pure indigo direct from its elements, and it will soon be a commercial product. Then the indigo fields, like the madder fields, will be abandoned, industrial laboratories having usurped their place.

Biochemists long ago advanced the theory that animal tissue is formed from the air inhaled, and not from food. The food, of course, serves its purpose- it acts as the negative pole, as does the earth to plant and vegetable life, and also furnishes the inorganic salts, the workers that carry on the chemistry of life, setting free magnetism, heat and electric forces by disintegration and fermentation of the organic portions of the food. But air, in passing through the various avenues and complex structure of the human organism, changes, condenses, solidifies, until it is finally deposited as flesh and bone. From this established scientific truth, it appears that, by constructing a set of tubes, pumps, etc., resembling the circulatory system, as well as the lung cells of the human mechanism, which is a chemical laboratory, where the chemistry of spirit is ever at work, changing the one essence of spirit substance to blood, flesh and bone, air may be changed into an albuminous pabulum, which may be again changed into the special kind of food required by adding the proper flavor, which may also be produced direct from the air.

There does not seem to be any reason why this substance, the basis of all food or vegetable growth, cannot, by proper process, be made into material for clothing. Wool, cotton, flax, silks, etc., are all produced from the universal elements through the slow, laborious and costly process of animal or vegetable growth. Why not produce them direct?

Those who believe in a time of peace on earth, a millennial reign, certainly do not think that our present mode of producing food will continue during that age. Slaughter of animals, and fruit, grain or vegetable raising leave small time for men and women to enjoy a condition foretold by all the seers and prophets. But under the new way of producing food and clothing, the millennium is possible.

And thus will the problem of subsistence be solved. No more monopoly of nature's bounties. An exchange of service will be the coin of the world instead of certain metals difficult to obtain. A realization of this vision, or theory, that will for awhile be called visionary by most people, will mean Eden restored. The Earth will be allowed to return to its natural state. We will cease to eat animals birds and fishes. Many people have wondered why, during the last few years fruit pests have multiplied so alarmingly, and why cows are almost universally diseased and so much attention given to meat, milk, and butter products by Boards of Health, etc. There is surely a reason. The One Life, Supreme Intelligence, or Divine Wisdom, that holds the worlds of space in their appointed orbits, surely knows all about the affairs of earth. When a new dispensation is about to be ushered in, old things begin to pass away.

All labor, preparing food and clothing, as now carried on, will cease, and the people, in governmental or collective capacity, will manufacture and distribute all manner of food and clothing free. Machinery for the production of everything necessary for man's material wants will be simple and easily manipulated. One-twentieth of the able-bodied population, working one or two hours a day, and shifting every week, or day, for that matter, with others, will produce an abundant supply. Neither droughts nor floods nor winter's snow can affect the supply. It can be made in Klondike or the Tropics. Garments may be worn for a few days and then burned, and laundry work cease. Cooking will be reduced to a minimum. No preparing vegetables, fruit or cracking nuts; no making butter, or preserving meats.

Men will not have to devote their lives to the endless grind of food production, nor women to cooking, dish-washing, sewing, and laundry-work. Garments of beautiful design and finest texture will be made by machines invented for the purpose, ready for wear. A dream, you say? I cannot admit that in the fact of the indisputable evidence already produced: but what if it were, at present, but the dream it may appear to the one who hears of its methods of operation for the first time? Do dreams ever come true? Yea, verily? All concrete facts are materialized dreams.

An Egyptian King dreamed, and the Pyramids of Cheops mass and miracle his vision. The Pyramids are encyclopedic of physical science and astral lore. The science of numbers, weights, measures, geometry astronomy, astrology, and all the deeper mysteries of the human body and soul are embodied in these incomparable monuments. A dream of an ancient alchemist solidified in stone, and the awful sphinx sat down in Egypt's sand to gaze into eternity. Columbus dreamed, and a white-sailed ship turned its prow west and west. On uncharted seas, with an eternity of water ahead, he remembered his dream, and answered "Sail on!" to the discouraged mate, until he landed on the unknown shores of a most wonderful new world. Michael Angelo dreamed a thousand dreams and sleeping marble awoke and smiled. Hudson and Fulton dreamed, and steamboats "run over and under the seas." The Pilgrim Fathers dreamed and America, the "marvel of nations" banners the skies with the stars and stripes. Marcus Whitman and Lewis and Clarke dreamed long and hard and the bones of oxen and men and women and

THE TREE OF LIFE

babies made a bridge over the desert sands and the mountain gorges to the shores of the Sundown Sea, and now the Pullman cars come safely over. Morse and Marconi and Edison dreamed strange wild dreams and concentrated intelligence springs from carbon-crucible and says to earth's boundaries, "Lo; here am I."

> Vibration of etheric substance
> Causing light through regions of space,
> A girdle of something enfolding
> And binding together the race
> And words without wires transmitted,
> Aerial-winged, spirit-sandaled and shod;
> Some call it electricity,
> And others call it GOD!

A mechanic dreamed, and sprang upon his automobile, and drove it till the axles blazed and the spaces shriveled behind him. Men of high strung airy brains dreamed wondrous dreams, and now the eagle's highway and the open road to men is parallel. A musician dreamed a sweet, harmonious dream, and forth from a throat of brass and discs of carbon directed by a million tiny fingers of steel, came the entrancing notes that had run riot through the singer's brain. So let us dream on, men and women, of the day of rest that is already dawning in the heavens. No wonder that Paul said:

"Now, brethren, are we the Sons of God, but it doth not yet appear what we shall be as such. The morning light of that glad day now purples the mountains of faith and hope with its rays of glory."

And when Man is once fully alive to his own heritage, realizing the wonders and possibilities of his own body, and to provide for its needs, he will assert the divine right within him to be an Ego, a soul, in command of its own temple, and the environments of that temple, and will rejoice in the revealed truth of his own divinity that alone can make him free.

PART TWO

The Bridge of Life

"A noiseless, patient spider,
I mark'd, where, on a little promontory, it stood, isolated;
Mark'd how, to explore the vacant, vast surrounding,
It launch'd forth filament, filament, filament, out of itself;
Ever unreeling them ever tirelessly speeding them.
And you, O my soul, where you stand,
Surrounded, surrounded, in measureless oceans of space,
Ceaselessly musing, venturing, throwing seeking the spheres, to
connect them;
Till the bridge you will need, be form'd till the ductile anchor hold;
Till the gossamer thread you fling, catch somewhere, O my soul."

-WALT WHITMAN

The statement by Holy Writ that "man is conceived in sin and brought forth in iniquity" has a threefold meaning, namely, chemical, physiological, and astrological. The translation from the Hebrew text as given is crude and misleading. The real meaning in the original is, that the human embryo remains nine months in the female laboratory, thus falling short three months of completing a solar year, or soul year.

THE TREE OF LIFE

Twelve represents a complete circle. The word sin comes from Schin, the 21st letter of the Hebrew alphabet, and means to fall short of completeness or understanding. In the Tarot symbol, S, or Sin, is represented by the "Blind Fool," one lacking in wisdom. "Brought forth in iniquity" is merely a repetition of the words "born in sin." Iniquity and inequity, or unequal, mean the same. The ancient Hebrews called Moon, Sin, because it gave light only part of the time.

To acquire wisdom that will enable the Ego in flesh to build a bridge across the three-month gap, or space between the point of conception and birth, is the one real problem that confronts Soul on the material plane of expression. The alchemists, seers, and astrologians of all ages have wrestled with this problem in their ceaseless endeavors to unravel the great mystery of man's dominion over flesh. Whether it be the chemist seeking new compounds, the physiologist searching and testing the fluids of the fearfully and wonderfully made body of man, or the alchemist probing for the Elixir of Life the Ichor of the Gods or the astrologian pulling and adjusting the etheric wires that criss-cross the spaces in an earnest desire to make good and sane the statement "The wise man rules his stars," all, all are seeking to span the awful space that yawns between the neophyte and the Promised Land of immortality in the body, where "in my flesh I shall see God," and when and where he can truly say with the regenerated Job, "I have heard of thee by the hearing of the ear, but now mine eye seeth thee." Man must work out his own salvation.

The bridge to be built across the three-months space must have a mineral base or rock foundation. "Thou are Peter (petra, stone, or mineral), on thee will I build my church," etc. Church is from the second Hebrew letter, Beth, a house, temple, or church. The human body is a house, temple, or church for Soul. "Know ye not that your bodies are the temple (church) of

THE TREE OF LIFE

God?" There are twelve inorganic mineral cell-salts in the human body, and these minerals (stones in the temple) correspond in vibration to the twelve signs of the Zodiac. During the nine months of gestation the embryo receives and appropriates the creative energies of nine of these salts, leaving three to be supplied after the parting of the umbilical cord. Take for example a native born February 22nd, with the Sun's entry into Pisces: The embryo having begun its journey at the gate of Gemini and negotiated the nine gestatory signs, his blood vibration at birth is thus deficient in the qualities of Pisces, Aries and Taurus, as also in the chemical dynamics of phosphate of iron, phosphate of potassium, and sulfate of sodium, the mineral bases respectively of the signs of this uncompleted quadrant. In so far as his circulatory system may receive these needed builders, health will be balanced and life prolonged.

The chemical union of these cell-salts with organic matter, such as oil, fibrin, albumen, etc., forms the various tissues of the body, and administers to the physiological needs as represented by the Bridge, that the multiple cells may respond more harmoniously and completely to the magic touch of the Divine energy, just as the tones of a musical instrument are made the more melodious through a properly skilled manipulation. And as bridge-building in a mechanical sense depends upon the plans and specifications of a competent civil engineer, so does the Bridge of Life depend upon the astrologian to chart and compass the way. Our diagram indicates at a glance the chemical formulas that appertain respectively to the zodiacal divisions, but to give a clearer conception as regards their specific qualities and physiological action in relation to the various signs, reference may be had to the following compend:

ARIES: From the teachings of the Chemistry of Life we find that the basis of brain or nerve fluid is a certain mineral salt known as potassium phosphate, or Kali Phos. The Phosphate of

24

THE TREE OF LIFE

Potash.

Synonyms: Potassium Phosphate, Kali Phosphoricum, Potassii Phosphas.

Formula: K_2HPO_4.

It may be prepared by mixing aqueous phosphoric acid with a sufficient quantity of potash, hydrate or carbonate, until the reaction is slightly alkaline and evaporating. Triturate to 3rd or 6th X. This salt is the great builder of the positive brain cells. Kali phos. unites with albumen and by some subtle alchemy transmutes it and forms gray brain matter. When the chemical possibilities of this brain builder are fully understood insane asylums will go out of fashion. Man has been deficient in understanding because his brain receiver did not vibrate to certain subtle influences; the dynamic cells in the gray matter of nerve were not finely attuned and did not respond hence sin, or falling short of understanding.

TAURUS: Sulfate of Soda.

Synonyms: Natrum Sulfate, Sodium Sulphuricum, Sodae or Sodii Sulphas, Glauber's Salts.

Formula: $Na_2 (SO_4 \ 10H_2O)$.

May be obtained by the action of Sulfuric acid on sodium chloride (common salt). This cell-salt is found in the intercellular fluids, liver and pancreas. Its principal work is to regulate the supply of water in the human organism. The blood becomes overcharged with water, either from the oxidation of organic matter or from inhaling air that contains more aqueous vapor (water) than is required to produce normal blood. This condition of air is liable to prevail whenever the temperature is above 70 degrees. One molecule of nat. sulph. has the power (chemical intelligence) to take up and carry away two molecules, or twice its bulk of water. The blood does not become overcharged with water from water taken into the stomach, but from the water lifted by expansion caused by heat above 70 degrees and held in the air and thus breathed into the arteries through the lungs. By the above we see that there is more work for this salt in hot weather than during cold weather. So-called malaria, Latin for bad air, is due to a lack of this tissue salt. Water lifted from swamps or clear streams or lakes by the action of the sun's heat is the same; for heat does not evaporate and lift poisonous disintegrating organic matter from a swamp or marsh, but the water only.

GEMINI: The Chloride of Potash, or Potassium.

Synonyms: Potassium chloride, Kali Muriaticum, Kali Chloratum, Kali Chloridum, Potassi Chloridum.

Formula: K Cl.

This salt must not be confused with the chlorate of potash, a poison, chemical formula K Clo3. Chloride of potash may be obtained by neutralizing pure aqueous hydrochloric acid with pure potassium carbonate or hydrate. The cell-salt kali muriaticum (Potassium chloride) is the mineral worker of blood that forms fibrin and properly diffuses it through the tissues of the body. Kali mur molecules are principal agents used in the chemistry of life to build fibrin into the human organism. The skin that covers the face contain the lines and angles that give expression and thus differentiate one person from another. In venous blood fibrin amounts to three in one thousand parts; when the molecules of Kali mur fall below the standard in the blood fibrin thickens, causing what is known as pleurisy, pneumonia, catarrh, diphtheria, etc. When the circulation fails to throw out the thickened fibrin via the glands or mucous membrane, it may stop the action of the heart. Embolus is a Latin word meaning little lump, or balls; therefore to die of embolus, or "heart failure" generally means that the heart's action was stopped by little lumps of fibrin clogging the auricles and ventricles of the heart. When the blood contains the proper amount of kali mur, fibrin is functional and the symptoms referred to above do not manifest.

CANCER: Fluoride of Lime.

Synonyms: Calcaria Flurica, Calcium Fluoride.

Chemical Formula: CaF_2.

This salt is formed by the union of lime and fluorine. The inorganic salts are the workers, controlled and directed by infinite intelligence, that performs the ceaseless miracle of creation or formation. Biologists and physiologists have searched long and patiently for a solution to the mystery of the differentiation of material forms. No ordinary test can detect any difference in the ovum of fish, reptile, bird, beast or man. Chemical analysis reveals the same mineral salts, carbon, oil, fibrine, albumen, sugar, etc., in the life cell, or ovum in the blood, tissue, hair, or bone of the multiple and varied expression of life in material forms. The chemistry of life answers the "Riddle of the Sphinx," and writes above the temple door of investigation: "Let there be light." There is no such thing as dead or inert. All is life. A crystal is an aggregation of living organism. The base of all material manifestation is mineral. "Out of the dust (ashes or mineral) of earth physical man is made." The twelve mineral salts of lime, iron, potash, sodium, silica and magnesium are the foundation stones of every visible form of animal or vegetable. No two forms of the different species of animals have the same combination of this "rock foundation," but all have some of the same minerals. It is quite as important for a student of Biochemistry to understand the process by which certain cell salts operate to supply a deficiency as it is to know what a particular symptom calls for. Elastic fiber, the chief organic substance in rubber, is formed by a chemical union of the fluoride of lime with albumen, oil, etc. Therefore, we find this salt dominant in the elastic fiber of the body, in the enamel of teeth and connective tissue. A lack of salt in proper amount causes relaxed condition of muscular tissue, falling of the womb and varicose veins. Sometimes there is a non-functional combination of this salt with oil and albumen which forms a solid deposit, causing swelling of stony hardness; it is a sort of incomplete fiber with other lime salts and vitiated fluids of the body.

LEO: Phosphate of Magnesia.

Synonyms: Magnesium Phosphorica.

Formula: MgHOPOJ (H2O).

This cell-salt may be made by mixing Phosphate of Soda with Sulfate of Magnesia. This salt is found chiefly in the white fibers of nerves and muscles. The tissues of nerves and muscles are composed of many very fine threads or strands of different colors, each acting as a special telegraph wire, each one having a certain conductive power or quality, special chemical affinity for, certain organic substances, oil or albumen, through and by which the organism is materialized and the process or operations of life are carried on. The imagination might easily conceive the idea that these delicate infinitesimal fibers are strings of the Human Harp, and that molecular minerals are the fingers of infinite Energy striking notes of some Divine Anthem. The white fibers of nerves and muscles need the dynamic action of Magnesia Phosphate especially to keep them in proper tune, or function, for by its chemical action on albumen the special fluid for white nerve or muscle fiber is formed. When the supply of this salt falls below the standard, cramps, sharp shooting pains or some spasmodic condition prevails. Such symptoms are simply calls of nature for more magnesia. The impulsive traits of Leo people are symbolized In the pulse, which is a reflex of heart throbs. The phosphate of magnesia, in biochemic therapeutics, is the remedy for all spasmodic impulsive symptoms. This salt supplies the deficient worker or builder in such cases and thus restores normal conditions. A lack of muscular force, or nerve vigor, indicates a disturbance in the operation of the heart cell-salt, magnesia phosphate, which gives the "Lion's spring," or impulse.

VIRGO: Sulfate of Potash.

Synonyms: Potassium Sulfate, Kali Sulphos, Potassae Sulphos, Kali Sulfate.

Formula: K_2SO_4.

The microscope reveals the fact that, when the body is in health, little jets of steam are constantly escaping from the seven million pores of the skin. The human body is a furnace and steam engine. The stomach and bowels burn food by chemical operation as truly as the furnace of a locomotive consumes by combustion. In the case of the locomotive the burning of coal furnishes force which vibrates water and causes an expansion (rate of motion) that we name steam. The average area of skin is estimated to be about 2,000 square inches. The atmospheric pressure being fourteen pounds to the square inch, a person of medium size is subject to a pressure of 40,000 pounds. Each square inch of skin contains 3500 sweat tubes or perspiratory pores (each of which may be likened to a little drain tile) one-fourth of an inch in length, making an aggregate length of the entire surface of the body 201,166 feet, or a tile draining for the body early forty miles in length. All tangible elements are the effects of certain rates of motion on the intangible and unseen elements. Nitrogen gas is mineral in solution, or ultimate potency. Oil is made by the union of the sulfate of potassium (potash) with albuminoids and aerial elements. The first element that is disturbed in the organism of those born in the celestial sign Virgo is oil; this break in the function of oils shows a deficiency in potassium sulfate, known in pharmacy as kali sulph. Virgo is represented in the human body by the stomach and bowels, the laboratory in which food is consumed as fuel to set free the minerals, in order that they may enter the blood through the mucous membrane absorbents. The letter X in Hebrew is Samech or Stomach. X or cross, means crucifixion, or charge, transmutation.

LIBRA: Phosphate of Soda.

Synonyms: Natrum Phosphate, Sodium Phosphate, Phosphos Natricus, Sodae Phosphate.

Formula: Na_2HPO_4; $12H_2O$.

This alkaline cell-salt is made from bone ash or by neutralizing orthophosphoric acid with carbonate of sodium. Sodium, or natrum, phosphate holds the balance between acids and normal fluids of the human body. Acid is organic and can be chemically split into two or more elements, thus destroying the formula that makes the chemical rate of motion called acid. Acid conditions are not due to an excess of acid in the blood, bile or gastric fluids. Supply the alkaline salt sodium phosphate, and acid will chemically change to normal fluids. A certain amount of acid is necessary, and always present in the blood, nerve, stomach and liver fluids. The apparent excess of acid is nearly always due to a deficiency in the alkaline, salt. Acid, in alchemical lore, is represented as Satan (Saturn), while sodium phosphate symbolizes Christ (Venus). An absence of the Christ principle gives license to Satan to run riot in the Holy Temple. The Advent of Christ drives the thief out with a whip of thongs. Reference to temple in the figurative language of Bible and New Testament always symbols the human organism. "Know ye not that your bodies are the Temple of the living God?" Solomon's temple is an allegory of the physical body of man and woman. Soul of man's temple the house, church, Beth or temple made without sound of "saw or hammer." Hate, envy, criticism, jealousy, competition, selfishness, war, suicide and murder are largely caused by acid conditions of the blood producing changes upon which Soul plays "Divine Harmonies" or "fantastic tricks before high heaven," according to the arrangement of chemical molecules in the wondrous laboratory of the soul. Without a proper balance of the alkaline salt, the agent of peace and love, man is fit for "treason, stratagem and spoils."

SCORPIO: Sulfate of Lime.

Synonyms: Calcium Sulfate, Calcarea Sulfate, Calc Sulphos, Gypsum, Plaster of Paris.

Formula: $CaSo_4$.

This salt can be obtained by precipitating a solution of chloride of lime with dilute sulfuric acid.

SAGITTARIUS : The mineral or cell-salt of blood corresponding to Sagittarius is Silica.

Synonyms: Silica, Silic, Oxide, White Pebble or Common Quartz. Chemical abbreviation, Si.

Made by fusing crude silica with carbonate of soda; dissolve the residue, filter, and precipitate by hydrochloric acid.

THE TREE OF LIFE

This product must be triturated as per biochemic process before using internally. This salt is the surgeon of the human organism. Silica is found in hair, skin, nails, periosteum, the membrane covering and protecting bone, the nerve sheath, called neurilemma, and a trace is found in bone tissue. The surgical qualities of silica lie in the fact that its particles are sharp cornered. A piece of quartz is a sample of the finer particles. Reduce silica to an impalpable powder and the microscope reveals the fact that the molecules are still pointed and jagged like a large piece of quartz rock. In all cases where it becomes necessary that decaying organic matter be discharged from any part of the body by the process of suppuration, these sharp-pointed particles are pushed by the marvelous intelligence that operates without ceasing, day and night, in the wondrous human Beth, and like a lancet cut a passage to the surface for the discharge of pus. Nowhere in all the records of physiology or biological research can anything be found more wonderful than the chemical and mechanical operation of this Divine artisan. The Centaur of mythology is known in the "Circles of Beasts that worship before the Lord (Sun) day and night," as Sagittarius, the Archer, with drawn bow. Arrow heads are composed of flint, decarbonized white pebble or quartz. Thus we see why silica is the special birth salt of all born in the Sagittarius sign.

CAPICORN: Phosphate of Lime.

Synonyms: Calcerea Phosphoricum, Calcium Phosphate. Formula: Ca3Po4.

Phosphoric acid dropped in lime water precipitates this salt. Circle means Sacrifice, according to the Cabala, the straight line bending to form a circle. Thus we find twelve zodiacal signs sacrificing to the sun. Twelve months sacrifice for a solar year. Twelve functions of man's body sacrifice for the temple, Beth, or "Church of God" the human house of flesh. Twelve minerals known as cell-salts sacrifice by operation and combining to build tissue. The dynamic force of these vitalized workmen constitutes the chemical affinities the positive and negative poles of mineral expression. The Cabalistic numerical value of the letters g, o, a, t, add up 12.

AQUARIUS: Sodium Chloride.

Synonyms: Natrum Muriaticum, Sodii Chloridium, Chloruretum, Chloruretum of Sodicum, Common table salt.

Must be triturated up to 3rd decimal before it can be taken up by mucous membrane absorbants and carried into the circulation.

Formula: NaCl.

Air contains 78 per cent of nitrogen gas, believed by scientists to be mineral in ultimate potency. Minerals are formed by the precipitation of nitrogen gas. Differentiation is attained by the proportion of oxygen and aqueous vapor (hydrogen) that unites with nitrogen. A combination of sodium and chlorine forms the mineral known as common salt. This mineral absorbs water. The circulation or distribution of water in the human organism is due to the chemical action of the molecules of sodium chloride. Aquarius is known as "The Water Bearer." Sodium chloride, known also as natrum muriaticum, is also a bearer of water, and chemically corresponds with the zodiacal angle of Aquarius.

PISCES: Phosphate of Iron.

Synonyms: Ferrum Phosphate, Ferri Phosphas.

Formula: $Fe_3 (PO_4)$

THE TREE OF LIFE

Phosphate of iron may be prepared by mixing sodium phosphate with sulfate of iron. The salt precipitated by this union is filtered, washed, dried and rubbed to a powder. The iron phosphate should not be used below the sixth (decimal trituration), as large doses of iron, as in tinctures, have a bad effect on the mucous lining of the stomach, injure the teeth and utterly fail to supply iron to the blood where it is needed to carry oxygen, the life giver. One red blood corpuscle does not exceed the one hundred and twenty millionth of a cubic inch. There are more than three million such cells in one drop of blood, and these cells carry the iron in the blood. How necessary, then, to administer the salts of iron to hungry cells in the most minute molecular form.

Each one of the twelve inorganic salts has its own sphere of function and curative action. Thus we find the phosphate of iron molecularly deficient in all fevers and inflammatory symptoms.

Health depends on a proper amount of iron phosphate in the blood, for the molecules of this salt have chemical affinity for oxygen and carry it to all parts of the organism. When these oxygen carriers are deficient, the circulation is increased in order to conduct a sufficient amount of oxygen to the extremities with the diminished quantity of iron, exactly as seven men must move faster to do the work of ten. This increased rate of motion of the blood is changed to heat, caused by friction, otherwise known as the "conservation of energy." This heat, or increase in the temperature of blood, has been named fever, from the Latin word fervere, meaning "To boil out."

The writer fails to see any relevancy between the word fever and a deficiency in iron phosphate molecules in the blood. From Hippocrates to Koch you will not find a true definition of fever outside of the Biochemic theory. It is not simply the heat that causes distress in a fever patient, but it is the lack of oxygen in the blood due to a deficiency in iron, the carrier of oxygen. The feet are the foundation of the body. Iron is the foundation of blood. Most diseases of Pisces people commence with symptoms indicating a deficiency of iron molecules in the blood; hence it is inferred that those born between the dates of February 19 and March 21 use more iron than do those born in other signs.

Iron is known as the magnetic mineral, due to the fact that it attracts oxygen. Pisces people possess great magnetic force "in their hands" and make the best magnetic healers. The astronomer, by the unerring law of mathematics applied to space, proportion, and the so far discovered wheels and cogs of the uni-machine, can tell where a certain planet must be located, before the telescope has verified the prediction. So the astrobiochemist knows there must of necessity be a blood mineral and tissue builder to correspond with each of the duodenary segments that constitute the circle of the Zodiac. Not through quarantine, nor disinfectants, nor boards of health, will man reach the long sought plane of physical well-being; nor by denials of disease will bodily regeneration be wrought; nor by dieting or fasting or "Fletcherizing" or suggesting, will the Elixir of Life and the Philosopher's Stone be found. The Mercury of the Sages and the "hidden manna" are not constituents of health foods. Victims of salt baths and massages are bald before their time, and the alcohol, steam and Turkish bath fiends die young. Only when man's body is made chemically perfect will the mind be able perfectly to express itself. And the secret of this chemical perfection is the sum total of the requirements involved in this zodiacal Bridge. The rock Peter, or Petra must be perfectly formed before the etheric wires which span the gulf between birth forward to the sidereal point of conception can vibrate in such harmony as to sustain the traveler on this "magical bridge of three piers," or the three zodiacal signs through which the material body must successfully function before it may hope to lift the veil of Isis.

The Bridge of Life, a symbol of physical regenesis, has been exploited in song, drama, and story. Paracelsus, Pythagoras, Lycurgus, Valentin, Wagner, and a long and unbroken line of the Illuminati, from time immemorial have chanted their epics in unison with this "riddle of the Sphinx," across the scroll of which is written, "Solve me, or die." Of all the multiple adepts or masters that have kept the lights burning above the Three Piers of the magical Bridge, none has more clearly and beautifully written thereof than did the great astrologian poet, Isaiah:

"Then the eyes of the blind shall be opened, and the ears of the deaf shall be unstopped. Then shall the lame man leap as a hart, and the tongue of the dumb shall sing; for in the wilderness shall waters break out, and streams in the desert. And the glowing sand shall become a pool, and the thirsty ground springs of water; in the habitation of jackals, where they lay, shall be grass with reeds and rushes. And a highway shall be there, and a way and it shall be called, The Way of Holiness; the unclean shall not pass over it, but it shall be for the redeemed; the wayfaring men, yea fools, shall not err therein."

PART THREE

Optic Thalmus

The inner eye "the eye behind the eye" just above and attached to the pineal gland by delicate electric wires, is called Optic Thalmus, and means "Light, or Eye of the Chamber."

In the Greek, it means "The Light of the World," "The Candlestick," "Wise Virgins," "The Temple Needs no Light of the Sun," "If Thine Eye be Single, Thy Whole Body shall be Full of Light," and other texts in the New Testament refer to the single eye or Optic Thalmus. Let us now search for the oil that feeds this wonderful lamp, the All-Seeing Eye.

Christ Jesus is made to say "I am the Light of the World." The word "world" comes from whirl," to turn as a wheel, to gyrate. The human body is a certain rate of activity, motion or whirl, IE. world, and the light of the world and the temple that needs no light of sun or moon refer to the body "Temple of God," when there is "oil in the lamp." Error is not sanctified by age. It behooves every lover of truth to cast aside prejudice and dogma and find truth. Until we know the meaning of the words "Jesus" and "Christ" we will not understand the bible, which was written in Greek and Hebrew and translated and retranslated to suit the whims and ignorance of priests and charlatans all down through the centuries. Constantine, a beast in human form, who murdered his mother and boiled his wife in oil, was the chief factor in the orthodox translation of the so-called King James bible.

Constantine was told by the priests of his time that there was no forgiveness of crimes like those that he was guilty of, and so this Roman Emperor devised the plan of salvation, in order that the blood of the innocent Jesus (or Christ) might save him from eternal damnation. An easy way out for this monster, and all the other blood-smeared tyrants, Kings, Emperors and Napoleons of finance, competition and war, from Pharaoh to the present day rulers whose thrones and scepters lie scattered and broken along the Highway of Nations (1917).

"Here the Vassal and the King, side by side, lie withering. Here the sword and scepter rust. "Earth to Earth, and dust to dust."

The word Jesus is from Ichtus, Greek for fish. The word

THE TREE OF LIFE

"Christ" means a substance of oil consistency, an ointment or smear. Varnish or paints are used to preserve or save wood or paper or cloth hence they become Saviors. At about the age of twelve, Jesus was found in the temple arguing with the doctors or teachers. The word "doctor" is from Latin "docere," to teach. Now read carefully: Every month in the life of every man or woman, when the moon is in the sign that the sun was in at the birth of the individual, there is a psycho-physical seed or "Son of Man" born near the Solar Plexus or the pneumo-gastric plexus which, in the ancient text, was called the "House of Bread," "The Tree of Life," etc. Bethlehem is from Beth, a house, and helm, bread. "Cast thy bread upon the waters and it shall return to thee after many days." Waters are the blood and nerve fluids of the body which carry the fish on its "Divine Journey" to regenerate, save and redeem man. Nazareth means to cook. Nazarene means cooked. Cook means to prepare. Any materialized thing is bread, Nazareth, mass, maso, or dough.

Thus the Catholic Mass. Also Maso-N. It will now be made plain why the Masons and Catholics are not in agreement, for our letter N is an abbreviation of the 14th letter of the Hebrew Alphabet, Nun, a fish. By adding N to Maso, the riddle of cooked or prepared fish was made so plain that the priesthood strenuously objected, and thus developed friction between the church and Masonry. The disciples were fishermen. The early Christians used a fish as their secret symbol. Money to pay taxes was taken from the mouth of a fish. Bread and fish were increased until 12 baskets full were left, etc. God prepared a fish to swallow Jonah.

Jonah means dove. Dove means peace the germ descending from the gray matter of the brain (See baptism of John). The storm means sex desire. The life seed was thus saved. "He that is born of God cannot sin (or fall short of knowledge) for his seed (fish) remaineth in him." John. The age of puberty is about 12. Up to that age, a child does not understand moral responsibility. "The first born" means the first seed or fish. Pharaoh, sex desire, always tries to destroy the first born. When Jesus was born in Bethlehem, he went (at the age of 12) up the pneumo-gastric nerve, which crosses the medulla oblongata at its junction with the spinal cord at the head of the "River of Jordan," the marrow or nerve fluid of the spinal cord (See illustration in Physiological Charts) and enters the cerebellum, the temple. This is the temple where the moral seed argued with the purely animal cells to change their rate of vibration to moral and spiritual concept. Later this seed (Jesus) drove those who bought and sold ("Even as you and I") with a whip of thongs out of the temple. We must all give up the animal life or suffer the same fate.

Before we explain the baptism in Jordan and the christening and the crucifixion, etc, let us briefly explain Moses, Joshua, Nile, Pharaoh and the children of Israel.

Egypt means the dark lower part of the body. That part of the body below the Solar Plexus is Egypt, or the Kingdom of Earth. All above the center, constitutes the Kingdom of Heaven. ("The Kingdom of Heaven is within you.") The Manger, or Bethlehem, is the center, or the balance. Nile, Moses and Pharaoh's daughter, all refer to generation. (See overflow of Nile). It rises in mountains of the moon. Moses means "drawn from the water." Fish are drawn from water. "There are two fishes in our sea" Vaughn. See Sign of Pisces, two fishes. Joshua the Son of Nun. Nun is Hebrew for fish. Moses was the physical or generative fish. Moses' laws were on the physical plane.

Joshua's laws were spiritual. Joshua means "God of Salvation," and salvation comes from saliva or salivation. Sal is salt which Saves. "If the salt loses its Savor" IE. Savior, wherewith shall it be salted?" Saliva saves the body by digesting (or preparing) the food. Saliva is a smear or ointment, and so

THE TREE OF LIFE

Joshua compares with Christ as Moses compared with Jesus. Moses died on Mt. Nebo. Nebo means understanding. Joshua took the place left vacant by the death of Moses. Jesus was baptized of John in Jordan the fluids, the Christ substance of the spinal cord, and became, "my beloved Son in whom I am well pleased." There is no J in the Greek or Hebrew alphabets, therefore, the word "John" I O H N meaning "Soul" or "fluids of the body" and not the Ego or Spiritual Man. So when the body dies, the fluids die thus man loses his soul when he loses his body. To prevent the loss of soul and flesh is the mission of the Son, or Seed, of God, or the Son of man.

There are two very small nerves that extend up from Solar Plexus, cross at base of brain and unite at the Optic Thalmus, the eye of the chamber. These nerves, or delicate wires, are called Adi and Pingali. After the seed or fish has been Christened, if it is retained and not wasted in sexual desire, it goes up to "Golgotha," the place of the skull, and crosses the wires, then remains three days in the tomb or the three chambers of the Pineal gland, then it enters the Optic Thalmus and "giveth light to all that are in the house," that is, the beth or body, all the twelve functions represented by the twelve disciples the twelve signs of the Zodiac. But the question will be asked What or where is the source or origin of this seed or redeeming Son? We answer: Ether, Spirit or God. Names mean nothing.

Esse, Universal intelligence, or It may be used. It breathes into man the breath of life. This elixir is carried through lungs into arteries, or air carriers, where it unites with the inorganic cell-salts, materializes (cooked), and forms granules, and is then deposited as flesh and bone. The study of Astrology, Biology and Biochemistry, added to Physiology, will lead one into the great Alchemical laboratory of the "Fearfully and wonderfully" made human temple the temple made without sound of saw or hammer.

THE TREE OF LIFE

Before the Neophyte can fully realize the power of the Optic Thalmus, the Divine Eye within his own brain, he must understand the meaning of Or especially in its relation to Word and Jordan.

Jordan (not Jordan) is the word in the original text. I is framed from Iod the 10th letter of the Hebrew Alphabet, and means "hand," or that which creates. Or is gold, not metal, but the "precious substance" the seed. Dan is Hebrew for Judge, therefore the Creative Power, operating through the precious substance, produces Judgment, or the man of good judgment. The upper brain is the reservoir of this Or and is the gray matter or "Precious Ointment" of Christ. "In the beginning was the Word and the Word was God. All things were (or is) created by it," etc. The upper brain is the Word, and it furnishes all that man contains, or is. Jesus was not a Savior until he was Christed of John in the Jordan. Then he became the "Beloved Son."

Why was the baptism necessary? Because there are two fish. One was Jesus, the Carpenter, the man; the other, the Christed Jesus the Son of God. The Christ substance gave the electric or magnetic power to the seed to cross the nerves at Golgotha without disintegrating or dying. To crucify, means to add to or increase a thousand fold. When electric wires are crossed, they set on fire all inflammable substances near them. When the Christed seed crossed the nerve at Golgotha, the veil of the temple was rent and there was an earthquake, and the dead came forth, IE. the generative cells of the body were quickened or regenerated. The crucifixion or crossing of the life seed gives power to vibrate the pineal gland at a rate that causes the Optic Thalmus to fill the "whole body with light," and send its vibration out along the optic nerve to the physical eye, and thus heal the blind. Let us hark back to the Nile: Pharaoh means a ruler or a tyrant or sex desire. Israel means blood, children of Israel, molecules of the blood. "Moses lifted up the serpent," etc.

41

THE TREE OF LIFE

Moses, the first born, the seed, desired to regenerate the blood and lead it to the promised land, thus he lifted up sex desire, here symbolized as the serpent (See the temptation of the Adam and Eve.) ... So shall the "Son of Man be lifted up," etc.. That is put on the cross in order to reach the pineal gland. "If I be lifted up, I will draw all men unto me, I will draw all other seed unto me. Study the etymology of "men."

The tree in the midst of the garden bore fruit every month and its leaves were healing. The Commandment to not eat of the fruit of this tree was not (is not) heeded by the race, and death is the result. The serpent said "Eat, thou shalt not die," but sex desire was a liar from the beginning. A noted Professor of Greek, in one of our Universities, says that the translation of many New Testament texts from Greek are radically wrong. For instance, "He that saveth his life, shall lose it, and he that loseth his life, for my sake, shall find it," should read: "He that saveth his seed life shall loosen it (set it free), and he that loosens it, shall find it," which means that this "Bread cast upon the waters" shall redeem him.

Galilee means a circle of water the fluids of the body. Jesus walking on the water is a symbol of the seed, or fish, on its journey. Peter, from petra (stone) is a symbol of physical or material thought which was rescued by the fish, Savior. The Optic Thalmus is called "The Lamb of God that taketh away the sins of the world" Sin is from the Hebrew letter Schin, meaning to fall short of knowledge. Sin does not mean wrong or crime, but one may commit a crime or do wrong through lack of knowledge. Paul said: "I die daily" ... "I am the chief of sinners." Revelations: "And the lamp thereof is the Lamb." The word, "Lamb," ends with B, which means a house or body of some kind. Now, the optic, or central single eye, is a body, like the outer eye ball; therefore, a beth. This is called lamb by the ancient poet.

THE TREE OF LIFE

Lamp ending with P, which means speech or sending forth or radiating, and is from Pe, the 8th letter of the Hebrew Alphabet, and was used to express light, or knowledge, emanating or going forth from this eye or "Lamb of God."

"As a man thinketh in his heart, so is he." The cerebellum is heart shaped, and in the Greek is known as the heart. The organ that divides blood was called the "Dividing Pump." The seat of thought is the Cerebellum. Our thoughts shape our lives. If we think continually below the solar plexus in the Kingdom of the Earth; if we dwell in thoughts of material pleasures, we become animal and materialistic. If we really desire the Kingdom of Heaven, we must think of the process that will enable us to realize it.

When Jesus was born, they put him in "swaddling clothes." Now the psychic germ (fish) is composed of the concentrated essence of life, and is covered by a gossamer capsule for protection. If this swaddling cloth is broken, the "precious ointment" is lost, i. e. it disintegrates and corrupts the blood. In order to save this germ of life, man must remember, that as a man thinketh, so is he. While men must abstain entirely from sexual contact, he must also realize that "He who looketh on a woman to lust after her, hath committed adultery with her in his heart"

By constant prayer do we attain the Kingdom. Envy, hatred, ambition, covetousness, will destroy the capsule that contains the seed, and thus corrupt the blood as surely as sexual contact. Alcohol in all its deceptive forms is the arch foe to this life-seed, and seeks by every means known to the enemy of man, to destroy it. "No drunkard shall inherit the Kingdom of Heaven," because alcohol destroys the redeeming substance that enables man to understand or think in his heart the thoughts of the Spirit. Alcohol cuts the capsule that holds the Esse, born

43

every month in Bethlehem. Alcohol eats the fruit of the tree of life. Gluttony is another enemy to regeneration. All excess of food, all that is not burnt up in the furnace the stomach and intestinal tract all that is not properly digested ferments and produces acid which develops alcohol. Auto intoxication is common among those who overeat. Most every one overeats.

The furnace, stomach and digestive tract, becomes a distillery, when the surplus food ferments; and thus becomes Babylon, the home of unclean birds and beasts which pander to carnal mind. Here we have the reason why sickness was considered Sin by the ancients: "To heal the sick and cast out devils" is the mission of the seed. "He that is born of God cannot sin, or be sick, for his seed remaineth in him." "The blood of Christ cleanseth from all sin"; therefore from all disease.

Here is the physiological explanation: When the Christed substance, the ointment from the river Jordan, the oil in the spinal cord, reaches the pineal gland, it vibrates to a rate that causes new blood the new wine. This is the blood of Christ that heals all infirmities. Unless, so-called, Christians repent of their sins, the doom of the church is at hand; "Mene, mene teckel upharsin" is written on the wall. Here are the words that define a Christian: "These signs shall follow those who believe; they shall lay hands on the sick and they shall recover. They shall cast out devils and raise the dead. All the things that I do, ye shall do, and greater things shall ye do."

If there be one Christian on Earth today, let him stand forth and prove himself worthy. "He that overcometh, I will give to eat of the fruit of the tree of life." To overcome a habit is to cease to do it. When the earthly man is controlled by the spiritual man the Lord God he ceases to eat of the fruit, that is, waste it. This fruit is then carried up to the brain and "Eaten in the Father's Kingdom." "And the last enemy to be overcome is death." We overcome death by ceasing to die, and in no other way. "He that believeth in me, shall not perish." Those who die are sinners, and, therefore, are not Christians, for Christ Jesus was (is) without sin. "The wages of Sin is death." "Repent, forsake evil, take up thy Cross, call upon the Lord and He will abundantly pardon." "And the ransomed of the Lord shall return and come to Zion."

When the sexual functions are used for the propagation of human bodies, there is no condemnation or sin. Motherhood is holy, pure, divine. But motherhood forced, is crime. Unwilling motherhood has created the spirit of war and murder and has well nigh destroyed the race. Sexual union for pleasure alone is the broad road that leads to death. "And there shall be no more Curse" (Revelation.) The word "Curse" has no reference to an oath. Curse means friction, to grind. The statement, "Then Peter began to curse and swear... And immediately the cock crew," when understood physiologically, fully explains the meaning of curse. Sexual commerce for the birth of children where the parents sacrifice themselves for their offsprings' sake, or total abstinence, is written with a pen of flame on all the pages of ancient Scriptures and modern biology.

"And I saw a woman clothed with the Sun, having the Moon under her feet and twelve stars upon her head." The Sun is the "Son of Man," the product of her own body saved and lifted up. The Moon refers to the generative life. Twelve stars are the twelve functions, typified by twelve zodiacal signs, which she has mastered through physical regeneration. Miss Ruth Le Prade, the woman poet of the New Time, sings of the Kingdom as follows:

"I am a woman free. My song
Flows from my soul with pure and joyful strength.
It shall be heard through all the noise of things

THE TREE OF LIFE

A song of joy where songs of joy were not.
My sister singers, singing in the past,
Sang songs of melody but not of joy
For woman's name was Sorrow, and the slave
Is never joyful, tho he smiles.

I am a woman free. Too long
I was held captive in the dust. Too long
My soul was surfeited with toil or ease
And rotted as the plaything of a slave.

I am a woman free at last
After the crumbling centuries of time.
Free to achieve and understand;
Free to become and live.

I am a woman free. With face
Turned toward the sun, I am advancing
Toward love that is not lust,
Toward work that is not pain,
Toward home which is the world,
Toward motherhood which is not forced,
And toward the man who also must be free.
With face turned toward the sun,
Strong and radiant-limbed,
I advance, singing,
And my song is as free
As the soul from which it flows.

I advance toward that which is, but was not;
I, the free woman, advance singing,
And with face turned toward the sun.
Let Ignorance and Tyranny
Tremble at the sound of my feet.

THE TREE OF LIFE

"When thou prayest, enter into thy closet and pray to thy Father in secret, and he shall reward thee openly." The word Secret is derived from Secretions. The upper brain, the Cerebrum, contains the secretions, gray matter, creative, or that creates, builds and supplies all life-force of the human temple. Soul of Man's (Solomon's temple). Hence God, the Creator, dwells in you. The cerebrum is his throne. Prayer or desires expressed by man in the cerebellum for righteousness, is answered in the cerebrum. Thus by prayer to God within, and in no other way, can man overcome the adversary or the "carnal mind which is at enmity to God." Let us now consider the Virgin Mary.

Virgin, pure. Mar-y, or mare, water. Virgin Mary, pure water. Pure Sea. Pure Ether or spirit. Fish come out of the water. The water, or fluids, of the body give birth to the seed, or fish. The Virgin Mary is not mentioned in the Allegory after the ascension of the Christed Jesus the redeemed fish. Each person, male or female, must "work out their own salvation." All so-called sex reform, that tolerates union of sexes, may be answered by:

"There is a way that seemeth right to man. The end of which is death."

"In my Kingdom there is no marrying nor giving in marriage, But they are as the Angels in Heaven."

Eden, good dwelling place, and Promised Land, mean the same. The children, molecules, of Israel, blood, crossed the Jordan in order to reach Eden. Jordan is the spinal cord, and the pneumo-gastric nerve crosses, at the junction of this cord, with the body known as Medulla oblongata, and thus connects with the cerebellum, which is the anteroom or Eden the head the "Thalmus" or chamber that contains the "Single Eye," the pineal

47

gland and upper brain or cerebellum. Eden's garden is the human body. The solar (center) plexus, with the pneumogastric plexus and its branches, is the "Tree of Life." The pneumo-gastric nerve is also called vagus nerve, beacuse its branches wander. Vagrant, wandering, is from vagus, to wander.

"A river went out of Eden to water the garden, and from thence it was parted and became four heads. The name of the first is Pishon; the second, Gihon; the third, Hiddekel; the fourth, Euphrates. The river is saliva. Pishon is the urine; Gihon is the intestinal tract; Hiddekel is the blood; Euphrates the nerve fluids, especially the creative. Abram and Sara, or Sarai, had the letter H added to their names when the angel appeared to them and gave instructions. See Gen. 16, 17 and 18. H is from Heth, the eighth letter of the Hebrew alphabet, and means a field or a vision. The meaning of Heth (H) is given in the Jewish Kaballa and Tarot card symbols as "Spiritual Perception" field, or vision. Sarah gave birth to Isaac after this regeneration. Isaac means laughter, a symbol of happiness; so the story is a symbol of physical regeneration.

The story of Job is evidently a fable. The letters I. O. B. (No J in Hebrew alphabet) figures up, numerically, 19, which means "resplendent light." Regeneration develops the optic thalmus, or single eye, by furnishing the oil necessary to light the chamber or Eden. "And the temple needs no light of Sun, Moon or Stars," etc. Job, on the generative plane, his experience in the Kingdom of Earth, suffered great trials, tribulations and disease; and while he argued much about God and kept his faith, he failed to comprehend. But after he became regenerated, he exclaimed:

"I have heard of thee by the hearing of the ear, but now mine eye seeth thee." Notice mine eye, not eyes.

So here we have another proof that regeneration opens

THE TREE OF LIFE

the Optic Thalmus the eye behind the eyes.

And now in closing:

No page of the wonders of the human body the temple of the living God is more divinely scientific than the parable that follows:

"The foolish man built his house on the sand And the rain washed it away."

"The wise man built his house on a rock And it stood the storms, for it was builded upon a rock."

The Bible is a compilation of astronomical, physiological and anatomical symbols, allegories and parables. In the technical terms of modern chemistry and physiology, the above text is explained as follows: Sand and cement form rock or stone. Sand alone, without some medium cement is unstable, simply "shifting sand." The Pineal gland, the dynamo that runs the organism of man, is composed of sand plus a cement, an ointment, a smear, found, as has been explained, in large quantity in the spinal cord, also, to some extent, in all parts of the body. When this cement is wasted, as the Prodigal Son wasted his substance in riotous living, there being a deficiency of this precious oil, the pineal gland becomes brittle, and does not vibrate at a rate that vitalizes the blood and tissue at the health and strength rate, and the house, beth or body, falls. In the common slang of the hour, we say: "He lacks the sand" or "grit."

The mineral salts of blood were called sand or salt by Hebrews. The cell-salts that are found in the pineal gland are chiefly potassium phosphate, the base of the gray matter of the brain; but all of the twelve inorganic salts are represented. In Revelations, the pineal gland is called "The white stone" In

49

THE TREE OF LIFE

Biochemistry, the phosphate of potassium is given as the birth-salts of Aries people. Those who build their house upon a rock are they who conserve the substance that unites with the sand cell-salts and thus forms the rock upon which a body may be built that will be free from sin and sickness. The mission of Jesus, the Christ, was to triumph over death and the grave, over matter, and transmute his body, and be able, also, to materialize at will. He not only succeeded in doing this, but stated most emphatically that all the things that he did, we may do also.

Did he proclaim the truth? Answer thou of little faith!

"Rock of Ages cleft for me,
Let me hide myself in thee."

And the Christ Substance shall create the cement that completes the rock surface of the bridge that crosses the three-span gulf between the shores of conception and birth. Thus "Shall Mortal put on immortality" and the last enemy, death, shall be overcome."

A VISION OF IMMORTALITY

It seemed to me that it was noon of a perfect day, and that I was wide awake. I stood upon a mountain top in Southern California and looked out to the West. I saw the clean page of the Balboa Sea.

Catalina Island reflected its hills and crags in the curling mists that rose and twisted about like things alive, and the mirage grew and spread until I fancied that the new Jerusalem was descending out of the Heavens.

Eastward the Sierra Madre peaks lightly veiled their

heads with mist and fleecy clouds, as if to gently subdue their ineffable glory. I saw the clean-trunked eucalypti, the pendant pepper boughs and the orange groves. A shuttle-throated mocking bird was pouring liquid melody into the ears of Deity, and I asked aloud, "Is not this immortality? Am I not immortal?" And then a voice, sweet as the voice of the Infinite Mother, came out of the everywhere, and I heard the words, "Yes! you are immortal. You stood in the rush of Divine Splendor when God said: 'Let there be light.' You heard the morning stars chant the Epic of Creation. You saw the first procession of the Constellations. You saw Orion light his clustering lamp out in the wilderness of the southern skies. You saw Arcturus rise from the unknown sea of silence, and sentinel the Northern Pole. You saw the first rushing, blazing Comet emerge from the awful realms of boundless space, sweep across measureless reaches of star-dust, bearing upon its flaming front the glad intelligence that the rule of law is perfect; that Suns, Stars, Systems obey the Cosmic urge and obey the Eternal Word. And, if in the operation of wisdom, the time shall come when the vast fabric of creation shall rock in universal spasm and totter to its fall, if the elements shall melt in fervent heat, the last Sun die and the 'Heavens be gathered together as a scroll,' yet thou, oh doubting one, shall stand erect, unafraid and;

> 'O'er the ruins smile
> And light thy torch again
> At Nature's funeral pile."

Then I heard the bugles all sing truce along the iron front of war. I saw the battle flags furled. Soldiers were transformed into men. They returned to homes, shops, the fields, the orchards and gardens. Children laughed and women loved. The headsman and hangman retired and became forgotten horrors. Grass grew over the battle trenches, flowers bloomed over deserted forts, vines clambered over arsenals and dreadnoughts rusted in the harbors. Earth was baptized with the golden light of love.

With the "Eye behind the eyes," "I saw the Holy City beside the tideless Sea" and I heard the Angels striking all their harps of gold.

THE END